Heart Manual

I0696911

A Clear Guide To Living Healthy

Sam Maxwell

Copyright

No part of this book should be copied, reproduced without the author's permission © 2023

Table Of Contents

INTRODUCTION

In the grand tapestry of human existence, the heart holds a position of profound significance. It is the ceaseless rhythm, the pulsating metronome, that orchestrates the symphony of life within us. This small, unassuming organ, nestled within our chest, is the linchpin of our vitality, tirelessly pumping life-giving blood through the intricate network of our circulatory system. Yet, amidst the cacophony of modern life, we often forget to pay homage to this tireless workhorse, to acknowledge its boundless dedication.

Heart Manual: A Clear Guide to a Healthy Heart is not just a book; it is an invitation to embark on a journey of understanding, nurturing, and safeguarding this vital organ. Within these pages, we delve deep into the realm of heart health, weaving together the threads of scientific knowledge, compassionate care, and actionable wisdom.

The Significance of Heart Health

The heart is more than a muscle; it is the very essence of our existence. Each beat propels life-giving oxygen and vital nutrients to every cell in our body. It is the silent sentinel that stands guard over our well-being, the sentinel we often take for granted. Yet, when the heart falters, when its rhythm stumbles, the repercussions echo through every aspect of our lives. Heart disease, a formidable adversary, knows no boundaries. It strikes the young and old, the robust and frail, without prejudice. Understanding and actively caring for our hearts is not just a matter of choice; it is a matter of necessity.

A Guide for All Ages

Heart Manual transcends age and circumstance. It is a compass for those navigating the ebullience of youth, a companion for those in the throes of midlife, and a beacon of hope for those savoring the wisdom of their golden years. The wisdom within these pages is for anyone who treasures life and recognizes the priceless value of health. It is for those seeking to fortify their heart health, for those who have witnessed the toll heart disease can take, and for those resolved to make changes that will resonate through the chambers of their hearts.

A Holistic Approach

This manual is more than a compilation of facts; it is a comprehensive guide, a repository of knowledge, and a source of empowerment. It will lead you through the intricate terrain of heart health, demystifying medical terminology and equipping you with practical tools to nurture and protect this vital organ. From comprehending the intricacies of the heart's anatomy to interpreting the language of symptoms, from making lifestyle choices that foster heart health to understanding the array of medical interventions available, each chapter is a stepping stone toward a stronger, healthier heart.

A Shared Journey

As you embark on this journey, know that you are not alone. We walk this path together, not just as a reader and a guide, but as fellow travelers on the road to a vibrant and heartful life. Your heart deserves nothing less than the utmost care and consideration, and together, we will explore the pathways to its well-being.

So, let us turn the page and begin this odyssey into the beating center of your existence. Welcome to Heart Manual: A Clear Guide to a Healthy Heart May it serve as the guiding light on your voyage to a heart filled with vitality and life.

Chapter 1

Understanding the heart

The heart, that silent sentinel nestled within our chests, is the unwavering conductor of life's symphony. To truly appreciate its significance, we must embark on a journey of understanding. This chapter is a gateway into the intricate world of the heart, an exploration of its anatomy, its ceaseless rhythm, and the orchestration of its vital functions. Here, we unravel the mysteries that lie beneath the surface, forging a deeper connection with this remarkable organ that sustains our existence. Join us as we delve into the beating center of our being, seeking to fathom the inner workings of the heart and gain a newfound appreciation for its boundless dedication.

Anatomy of the heart

The heart, a marvel of biological engineering, is a muscular organ that serves as the epicenter of the circulatory system. Nestled within the protective embrace of the ribcage, it beats with rhythmic precision, tirelessly pumping life-sustaining blood to every corner of the body. To truly grasp the complexity and wonder of this vital organ, one must embark on a journey through its intricate anatomy.

External Structure:

The heart, roughly the size of a clenched fist, is positioned in the thoracic cavity, slightly to the left of the sternum. It divided into four chambers, two atria and two ventricles. The exterior surface is encased in a double-layered sac known as the pericardium, which not only provides protection but also allows the heart to move within the chest with minimal friction.

Chambers of the Heart:

The heart's four chambers play distinct yet interdependent roles in the circulation of blood. The right atrium receives deoxygenated blood returning from the body's various tissues, while the left atrium receives oxygen-rich blood from the lungs. These atria serve as reservoirs, allowing blood to flow into the ventricles below.

Beneath the atria lie the ventricles, where the real work of the heart takes place. The right ventricle pumps deoxygenated blood into the pulmonary artery, which leads to the lungs for oxygenation. Simultaneously, the left ventricle, endowed with formidable muscularity, propels oxygenated blood into the aorta, the body's largest artery, initiating the journey to nourish cells, tissues, and organs.

Valves:

Within the heart lie a set of remarkable valves that ensure unidirectional blood flow. The tricuspid valve guards the passage between the right atrium and right ventricle, while the bicuspid or mitral valve separates the left atrium from the left ventricle. These valves open and close in synchrony with the heart's contractions, preventing backflow and maintaining the integrity of circulation.

At the exit points of the ventricles, two more valves reign. The pulmonary valve guards the exit of the right ventricle into the pulmonary artery, directing blood towards the lungs. On the left side, the aortic valve controls the flow from the left ventricle into the aorta, channeling oxygen-rich blood into the systemic circulation.

The Coronary Circulation:

The heart, despite its tireless work, is not exempt from its own metabolic demands. This is met by the coronary circulation, a network of blood vessels that supply the heart muscle itself. The coronary arteries branch off from the aorta, encircling the heart and ensuring it receives the oxygen and nutrients it requires to continue its rhythmic duty.

Conclusion:

The anatomy of the heart is a testament to nature's ingenuity. Its meticulous design, from chambers and valves to arteries and veins, ensures the seamless flow of life itself. Understanding this intricate orchestration is not only a journey through science, but an appreciation of the awe-inspiring symphony that sustains us. As we delve into the depths of the heart's anatomy, we gain a profound reverence for this remarkable organ that beats in rhythm with our very existence.

How The Heart Works

The heart, a tirelessly beating marvel, is the linchpin of the circulatory system, orchestrating a symphony of life within our bodies. It operates with a precision that rivals the finest timepiece, ensuring that oxygenated blood reaches every cell and that waste products are efficiently removed. To comprehend the marvel of this rhythmic conductor, we must delve into the mechanics that drive its ceaseless motion.

The Cardiac Cycle:

The heart's operation can be likened to a cycle, a rhythmic sequence of events that repeats with each beat. This cycle is divided into two main phases: systole and diastole. During systole, the heart contracts, pushing blood out into the circulatory system. Conversely, diastole is the relaxation phase, allowing the heart to fill with blood in preparation for the next cycle.

Atrial Contraction and Ventricular Filling:

The cycle begins with a gentle nudge from the sinoatrial (SA) node, the heart's natural pacemaker, located in the right atrium. The SA node initiates an electrical impulse that spreads across the atria, causing them to contract. This contraction propels blood into the ventricles.

Simultaneously, the atrioventricular (AV) node, positioned at the junction between the atria and ventricles, momentarily delays the electrical signal. This delay ensures that the atria have ample time to empty their contents into the ventricles before they contract.

Ventricular Contraction and Atrial Relaxation:

Once the ventricles are adequately filled, the electrical impulse descends to the atrioventricular bundle (Bundle of His), a specialized conducting pathway. This bundle then branches into Purkinje fibers, which rapidly disseminate the signal throughout the ventricles. This coordinated electrical stimulation leads to a powerful contraction of the ventricles, forcing blood into the pulmonary artery from the right ventricle and into the aorta from the left ventricle.

Simultaneously, the atria are in a state of relaxation, allowing them to refill with blood from the veins in preparation for the next cycle.

Valves: Guardians of Unidirectional Flow:

Critical to the heart's function are its valves, guardians that ensure blood flows in one direction. The tricuspid and bicuspid (mitral) valves separate the atria from the ventricles, preventing backflow. Likewise, the pulmonary and aortic valves guard the exits from the ventricles, allowing blood to be propelled into the arteries while preventing regurgitation back into the ventricles.

The Circulatory Dance:

As the heart contracts, oxygen-rich blood is propelled into the aorta and pulmonary arteries, initiating a journey that spans the entire body. The arteries, like tributaries branching from a river, carry blood to tissues and organs, nourishing them with oxygen and nutrients. Meanwhile, veins return deoxygenated blood and waste products back to the heart, completing the circulatory loop.

Conclusion:

The heart's rhythmic ballet of contraction and relaxation, guided by a finely-tuned electrical system, sustains us from the first beat to the last. Understanding this intricate interplay of anatomy and physiology is to grasp the essence of life itself. It is a testament to the remarkable design of nature, a symphony of vitality that echoes through our every moment.

As we delve into the mechanics of the heart, we gain not only knowledge but a profound appreciation for this ceaseless conductor that keeps the rhythm of our existence alive

Common Hearth Condition

1. Coronary Artery Disease (CAD):

Overview:Coronary artery disease is a condition characterized by the narrowing or blockage of coronary arteries, the vessels that supply oxygen-rich blood to the heart muscle. This is primarily due to the build-up of plaque, a combination of cholesterol, fat, and other substances.

Symptoms:Chest pain (angina), shortness of breath, fatigue, and in severe cases, heart attacks.

Treatment: Lifestyle changes (diet, exercise, smoking cessation), medications, angioplasty, stent placement, or bypass surgery in advanced cases.

2. Heart Failure:

Overview:Heart failure occurs when the heart is unable to pump blood efficiently to meet the body's demands. It can result from various conditions, including CAD, high blood pressure, or heart valve disorders.

Symptoms:Fatigue, shortness of breath, swelling in the legs and ankles, and fluid retention.

Treatment: Medications (diuretics, ACE inhibitors, beta-blockers), lifestyle changes, heart-healthy diet, and, in severe cases, heart transplant.

3. Arrhythmias:

Overview: Arrhythmias are irregular heart rhythms, either too fast (tachycardia) or too slow (bradycardia), which disrupt the heart's normal electrical signaling.

Symptoms:Palpitations, dizziness, chest discomfort, and in severe cases, fainting.

Treatment: Medications, electrical cardioversion, catheter ablation, or the implantation of a pacemaker or defibrillator.

4. Valvular Heart Disease:

Overview:This condition arises when the heart's valves, which regulate blood flow, become damaged or dysfunctional. It can involve stenosis (narrowing) or regurgitation (leakage) of the valves.

Symptoms: Fatigue, shortness of breath, chest pain, and palpitations.

Treatment: Medications, valve repair or replacement surgery, or minimally invasive procedures like TAVR (Transcatheter Aortic Valve Replacement).

5. Hypertension (High Blood Pressure):

Overview: Hypertension is a chronic condition characterized by elevated blood pressure levels, which can strain the heart and blood vessels over time.

Symptoms: Often asymptomatic, but can lead to headaches, fatigue, chest pain, and in severe cases, organ damage.

Treatment: Lifestyle modifications (diet, exercise, stress management), medications, and regular monitoring.

6. Cardiomyopathy:

Overview: Cardiomyopathy refers to a group of diseases that weaken the heart muscle, reducing its ability to pump blood effectively.

Symptoms: Fatigue, swelling in the legs, shortness of breath, and irregular heart rhythms.

Treatment:Medications, lifestyle changes, implantable devices (pacemakers, defibrillators), and in severe cases, heart transplant.

7. Congenital Heart Defects:

Overview:These are structural abnormalities in the heart present at birth. They can involve issues with the heart's walls, valves, or blood vessels.

Symptoms:Vary widely depending on the specific defect, ranging from mild to severe.

Treatment:

Medications, catheter-based interventions, open-heart surgery, or heart transplant, depending on the nature and severity of the defect.

Conclusion:

Understanding these common heart conditions is pivotal in maintaining heart health. Early recognition of symptoms and appropriate medical intervention can greatly improve outcomes.

Regular check-ups, a heart-healthy lifestyle, and prompt attention to any concerning signs are essential steps in preserving the vitality of this remarkable organ that sustains our lives.

Chapter 2

Assessing your heart health

Assessing heart health is a fundamental step towards maintaining overall well-being and longevity. A healthy heart is the cornerstone of a thriving life, as it ensures optimal circulation of oxygen-rich blood to every part of the body. This introductory process involves a comprehensive evaluation of various vital indicators, ranging from blood pressure and cholesterol levels to lifestyle habits and genetic predispositions. By understanding and actively managing these factors, individuals can take proactive steps towards reducing the risk of cardiovascular diseases, enhancing their quality of life, and promoting a vibrant, heart-healthy future. This introductory assessment serves as the cornerstone for a holistic approach to heart health, empowering individuals to make informed choices that can positively impact their cardiovascular well-being.

Risk Factors For Heart Disease

1. High Blood Pressure (Hypertension): Elevated blood pressure puts extra strain on the heart and arteries, leading to the development of heart disease over time. It is one of the most significant risk factors for heart disease.

2. High Cholesterol: High levels of LDL (low-density lipoprotein) cholesterol in the blood can lead to the buildup of fatty deposits (plaques) in the arteries, a condition known as atherosclerosis. This narrows the arteries and restricts blood flow to the heart.

3. Smoking: Cigarette smoking is a major risk factor for heart disease. The chemicals in tobacco can damage the heart and blood vessels, and also contribute to the development of atherosclerosis.

4. Diabetes: Both type 1 and type 2 diabetes increase the risk of heart disease. High blood sugar levels can damage the arteries and lead to atherosclerosis. Additionally, people with diabetes are more likely to have other risk factors like high blood pressure and high cholesterol.

5. Obesity and Overweight: Carrying excess weight, especially around the abdomen, increases the risk of heart disease. Obesity is associated with conditions like high blood pressure, high cholesterol, and diabetes, all of which contribute to heart disease.

6. Physical Inactivity: Lack of regular physical activity is a significant risk factor for heart disease. Exercise helps maintain a healthy weight, lower blood pressure, and improve cholesterol levels.

7. Unhealthy Diet: A diet high in saturated and trans fats, cholesterol, and sodium can contribute to the development of heart disease. It can lead to high cholesterol levels, high blood pressure, and obesity.

8. Family History and Genetics: If close family members (parents or siblings) have had heart disease, your risk is increased. Some genetic factors can also predispose individuals to heart disease.

9. Age: The risk of heart disease increases with age. Men over 45 and women over 55 are at higher risk. This is partly because arteries tend to narrow and become less flexible as we age.

10. Gender: Men are generally at higher risk of heart disease at a younger age, but women's risk increases after menopause. This is due, in part, to hormonal changes.

11. Stress: Chronic stress can contribute to heart disease, although the exact mechanisms are not fully understood. It may lead to unhealthy coping mechanisms such as overeating, smoking, or excessive alcohol consumption.

12. Excessive Alcohol Consumption: Heavy and regular alcohol consumption can lead to high blood pressure, heart failure, and other heart-related problems.

13. Sleep Apnea: This sleep disorder is associated with an increased risk of high blood pressure, which is a major risk factor for heart disease.

It's important to note that while these factors increase the risk of heart disease, they do not guarantee its development. Many people with multiple risk factors never develop heart disease, while some with few or no apparent risk factors do. Lifestyle modifications, regular health check-ups, and early intervention can significantly reduce the risk of heart disease. If you have concerns about your heart health, it's best to consult a healthcare professional.

Family History And Genetics

Family history and genetics play a crucial role in assessing an individual's risk for heart disease. They provide valuable information about inherited traits and predispositions that can influence cardiovascular health. Here's an extensive look at how family history and genetics contribute to understanding and managing heart health:

1. Inherited Risk Factors:

Genetic Mutations: Certain genetic mutations can directly impact the structure and function of the heart, leading to conditions like hyper trophic cardiomyopathy, familial hypercholesterolemia, and arrhythmias.

-Polygenic Risk: Heart disease is influenced by multiple genes, each with a small effect. Analyzing a person's genetic profile can help estimate their overall genetic risk for heart disease.

2. Familial Clustering:

- When multiple close relatives (such as parents or siblings) have a history of heart disease, it suggests a potential genetic predisposition within the family.

- The more close relatives affected, and the younger they were when diagnosed, the higher the familial risk.

3. Early Onset of Heart Disease:

- If a family member experienced heart disease at an early age (before 55 in men and before 65 in women), it may indicate a stronger genetic influence.

4. Specific Cardiovascular Conditions:

- Different heart conditions may have distinct patterns of inheritance. For example, some forms of cardiomyopathy or arrhythmias have a strong genetic component.

5. Shared Lifestyle and Environmental Factors:

- Families often share similar lifestyles, including dietary habits, exercise routines, and exposure to environmental factors like secondhand smoke or pollutants. These commonalities can contribute to familial heart health patterns.

6. Genetic Testing:

- Advances in genetic testing allow for the identification of specific genetic variations associated with increased risk of heart disease. This can be particularly relevant for conditions like familial hypercholesterolemia.

7. Risk Modification and Prevention:

- Knowing about a family history of heart disease can motivate individuals to adopt a healthier lifestyle and seek regular medical check-ups. This proactive approach can help in early detection and management of risk factors.

8. Tailored Screening and Monitoring:

- Individuals with a significant family history of heart disease may benefit from more intensive screening protocols, including more frequent blood pressure measurements, cholesterol checks, and cardiac evaluations.

9. Risk Communication:

- Understanding one's family history of heart disease allows for informed discussions with healthcare providers. It helps in devising personalized prevention and treatment plans.

10. Psycho social Impact:

- Being aware of a family history of heart disease can have emotional and psychological implications. It may serve as a motivator for positive lifestyle changes, or it could cause heightened anxiety, warranting appropriate support and counseling.

11. Genetic Counseling:

- In cases where a specific genetic mutation is identified, genetic counseling can provide valuable information about the inheritance pattern, potential risks for offspring, and options for preventive measures.

12. Research and Future Developments:

- Family history and genetic information contribute to ongoing research on the genetic basis of heart disease. This research informs the development of targeted therapies and interventions.

It's important to note that while genetics and family history are significant factors, they interact with lifestyle and environmental influences. Making positive lifestyle choices, such as maintaining a balanced diet, engaging in regular exercise, avoiding smoking, and managing stress, remains essential in reducing the overall risk of heart disease. Consulting with a healthcare provider or genetic counselor can help individuals understand their specific risk profile and develop a tailored approach to heart health.

Chapter 3

Maintaining a heart healthy lifestyle

Maintaining a heart-healthy lifestyle is the cornerstone of promoting cardiovascular well-being and reducing the risk of heart disease. A balanced approach encompassing dietary choices, regular exercise, stress management, and prudent lifestyle decisions can significantly enhance the health and functionality of your heart. By adopting these practices, you empower yourself with the tools to safeguard one of your body's most vital organs, ensuring it functions optimally for a long and vibrant life. This comprehensive guide will delve into various aspects of a heart-healthy lifestyle, offering practical tips and insights to help you make informed choices for your cardiovascular well-being.

Balance diet for heart health

Maintaining a balanced diet is paramount for heart health. A well-rounded and nutritious diet can help control risk factors such as high blood pressure, high cholesterol levels, and excess body weight, all of which are associated with heart disease. Here is an extensive guide on a balanced diet for heart health:

1. Fruits and Vegetables:

  - Include a large variety of colorful fruits and vegetables in your diet. They are rich in vitamins, minerals, antioxidants, and fiber. Aim for at least 5 servings per day.

2. Whole Grains:

  - Opt for whole grains like brown rice, whole wheat bread, quinoa, oats, and whole grain pasta. These are rich in fiber, which helps regulate cholesterol levels and promote heart health.

3. Lean Proteins:

  - Prioritize lean sources of protein, such as poultry, fish, legumes (beans, lentils, chickpeas), tofu, and low-fat dairy products. Limit consumption of red and processed meats, which can increase cholesterol levels.

4. Fatty Fish:

- Include fatty fish like salmon, mackerel, sardines, and trout in your diet. They are high in omega-3 fatty acids, which have been shown to lower triglycerides, reduce inflammation, and support heart health.

5. Nuts and Seeds:

- Almonds, walnuts, flax seeds, chia seeds, and sunflower seeds are rich in heart-healthy fats, fiber, and various nutrients. They can help lower cholesterol levels and improve overall cardiovascular health.

6. Healthy Fats:

- Incorporate sources of unsaturated fats like avocados, olive oil, and olives. These fats have been associated with a reduced risk of heart disease when consumed in moderation.

7. Dairy and Alternatives:

- Choose low-fat or fat-free dairy products like milk, yogurt, and cheese. Alternatively, opt for fortified plant-based alternatives like almond milk or soy milk, which can be lower in saturated fat.

8. Limit Saturated and Trans Fats:

- Minimize consumption of foods high in saturated and trans fats, such as fried foods, pastries, and commercially baked goods.

These fats can raise cholesterol levels and contribute to heart disease.

9. Limit Added Sugars and Refined Carbohydrates:

- Reduce intake of sugary beverages, candies, and desserts. Opt for whole fruits over fruit juices and choose complex carbohydrates over refined ones.

10. Limit Sodium Intake:

- Avoid excessive salt by using herbs and spices to flavor your food. Read food labels to identify high-sodium products and opt for lower sodium alternatives.

11. Portion Control:

- Be mindful of portion sizes to stop overeating. Proper portion control helps maintain a healthy weight and supports heart health.

12. Hydration:

- Stay well-hydrated by drinking an adequate amount of water daily. Proper hydration supports overall bodily functions, including cardiovascular health.

13. Moderate Alcohol Consumption:

- If you want to drink alcohol, do so in moderation. For men, this typically means up to two drinks per day, and for women, up to one drink per day.

14. Balanced Meal Planning:

- Aim for balanced meals that incorporate a combination of carbohydrates, proteins, and healthy fats. This helps stabilize blood sugar levels and provides sustained energy throughout the day.

15. Limit Processed and Fast Foods:

- Minimize consumption of processed and fast foods, as they are often high in unhealthy fats, sodium, and added sugars.

By adopting a balanced diet rich in whole, nutrient-dense foods, you provide your body with the essential nutrients it needs to support optimal heart health. It's important to remember that consistency in making healthy food choices is key, and consulting with a healthcare provider or registered dietitian can provide personalized guidance based on your specific health needs and goals.

Exercise and physical activities

Exercise and physical activity are fundamental components of a healthy lifestyle, contributing to overall well-being and reducing the risk of various chronic diseases, including heart disease, obesity, and diabetes. Here's an extensive guide on exercise and physical activities:

1. Types of Exercise:

- Cardiovascular (Aerobic) Exercise: This type of exercise increases your heart rate and breathing rate. It includes activities like brisk walking, jogging, cycling, swimming, dancing, and aerobics classes.

- Strength Training (Resistance) Exercises: These activities focus on building muscle strength and endurance. This can be done using weights, resistance bands, or body weight exercises like push-ups and squats.

- Flexibility and Stretching Exercises: Stretching exercises help improve flexibility and range of motion. They include activities like yoga, Pilates, and specific stretching routines.

- Balance and Stability Exercises: These activities help improve balance and coordination, which are crucial for preventing falls, especially in older adults. Examples include tai chi and specific balance exercises.

2. Frequency and Duration:

- Aim for at least 150 minutes of moderate-intensity aerobic activity or 75 minutes of vigorous-intensity activity per week, as recommended by health authorities. This can be broken down into sessions of 30 minutes, five days a week, or adjusted according to individual preferences and fitness levels.

- Incorporate strength training exercises for all major muscle groups on at least two days a week.

3. Progression and Variation:

- Gradually increase the intensity, duration, or frequency of your workouts to challenge your body and continue making progress. This can be achieved by adding more weight, increasing speed, or trying new activities.

4. Flexibility and Stretching:

- Include stretching exercises in your routine to improve flexibility and reduce the risk of injury. Stretch before and after your workouts to enhance range of motion and prevent muscle stiffness.

5. Warm-up and Cool-down:

- Always begin your exercise session with a warm-up to prepare your body for more intense activity. Likewise, end with a cool-down period to gradually lower your heart rate and ease your body back to a resting state.

6. Safety and Form:

- Prioritize proper form and technique to prevent injuries. If you're unsure about how to perform an exercise, seek guidance from a qualified fitness professional.

7. Listen to Your Body:

- Pay attention to how your body feels during exercise. If you experience pain, dizziness, or extreme fatigue, stop and seek medical advice if necessary.

8. Consistency is Key:

- Regular, consistent exercise is more beneficial than sporadic intense workouts. Find activities you enjoy and make them a regular part of your routine.

9. Adapt to Your Lifestyle:

- Fit exercise into your daily life. This can include walking or biking to work, taking the stairs, or incorporating physical activities into social events.

10. Stay Hydrated:

- Drink water before, during, and after exercise to stay properly hydrated. Dehydration can negatively impact performance and recovery.

11. Incorporate Fun and Variety:

- Choose activities you enjoy to make exercise a pleasurable part of your life. This could be dancing, hiking, playing sports, or trying new fitness classes.

12. Consult a Healthcare Professional:

- If you have any existing health conditions or concerns, consult with a healthcare provider before starting a new exercise program. They can provide tailored advice based on your specific needs.

13. Rest and Recovery:

- Allow your body adequate time to rest and recover between workouts. This is when your muscles repair and strengthen, leading to improved fitness levels.

14. Set Realistic Goals:

- Establish achievable, specific goals to track your progress and stay motivated. Whether it's running a certain distance, lifting a certain weight, or improving flexibility, setting targets can provide a sense of accomplishment.

Remember, the most effective exercise routine is one that you enjoy and can maintain over the long term. It's not about perfection, but about making consistent, sustainable efforts to improve your overall physical health and well-being.

Stress Management Techniques

management. Managing stress is crucial for heart health, as chronic stress can contribute to high blood pressure, inflammation, and other cardiovascular issues. Here are some extensive techniques for stress management to help support a heart-healthy lifestyle:

1. Regular Exercise: Engaging in regular physical activity is one of the most effective ways to manage stress and promote heart health. Exercise releases endorphins, which are known as "feel-good" hormones that can help alleviate stress and develop mood. Aim for at least 150 minutes of moderate-intensity exercise per week, such as brisk walking, jogging, swimming, or cycling.

2. Deep Breathing and Relaxation Techniques: Deep breathing exercises like diaphragmatic breathing, progressive muscle relaxation, and guided imagery can help calm the nervous system and reduce stress levels. These techniques can be practiced daily or during particularly stressful moments.

3. Meditation and Mindfulness: Mindfulness meditation involves paying focused attention to the present moment without judgment. Regular practice can improve emotional regulation and reduce stress. Apps like Headspace and Calm can be helpful for guided meditation sessions.

4. Yoga: Yoga combines with physical postures, breathing exercises, and meditation to promote relaxation and reduce stress. It also enhances flexibility, strength, and balance, which contribute to overall heart health.

5. Adequate Sleep: Getting enough restorative sleep is crucial for both stress management and heart health. Aim for 7-9 hours of good sleep per night. Establishing a regular sleep routine, creating a comfortable sleep environment, and avoiding stimulants like caffeine before bedtime can help improve sleep quality.

6. Balanced Diet: Eating a heart-healthy diet rich in fruits, vegetables, whole grains, lean proteins, and healthy fats can help regulate blood pressure, cholesterol levels, and overall heart function. Avoiding excessive consumption of processed foods, sugary snacks, and high-sodium foods is also important.

7. Limiting Caffeine and Alcohol: Both caffeine and alcohol can impact sleep quality and increase stress levels if consumed in excess. Moderation is key, and it's advisable to limit these substances, especially in the hours leading up to bedtime.

8. Social Support and Connection: Maintaining strong social connections with family and friends provides emotional support and can help alleviate stress. Spending quality time with loved ones and engaging in activities that foster positive social interactions are important for mental well-being.

9. Time Management and Prioritization: Effective time management can help reduce the feeling of being overwhelmed and stressed. Setting realistic goals, prioritizing tasks, and avoiding overcommitting can contribute to a more balanced and less stressful lifestyle.

10. Seeking Professional Help: If stress becomes chronic or overwhelming, seeking help from a mental health professional, such as a therapist or counselor, can provide valuable support and coping strategies.

Remember, it's important to individualize these techniques to suit your preferences and lifestyle. Consistency is key, and incorporating these practices into your daily routine can contribute to a healthier, happier, and more heart-healthy life. Always consult with a healthcare professional before making significant changes to your exercise or diet regimen, especially if you have underlying health conditions.

Adequate Sleep And Rest

Adequate sleep and rest play a crucial role in maintaining a healthy heart lifestyle. Here are some extensive points explaining this:

1.Regulates Blood Pressure: Getting enough sleep helps regulate blood pressure. Chronic sleep deprivation can lead to elevated blood pressure levels, which is a risk factor for heart disease.

2.Reduces Stress Levels: Quality sleep contributes to lower stress levels. When you're well-rested, your body produces lower levels of stress hormones like cortisol. High stress levels are associated with an increased risk of heart disease.

3. Balances Hormones: Sleep is essential for the regulation of various hormones in the body. This includes hormones like insulin, which is crucial for blood sugar regulation. Poor sleep can lead to insulin resistance, which is a risk factor for heart disease.

4.Promotes Healthy Weight: A well-rested body is more likely to maintain a healthy weight. Sleep deprivation disrupts the balance of hunger-regulating hormones (ghrelin and leptin), leading to increased appetite, particularly for high-calorie, sugary foods. This can contribute to weight gain and obesity, both of which are associated with heart disease.

5.Improves Immune Function: Quality sleep strengthens the immune system, enabling the body to better fight off infections and inflammation. Chronic inflammation is a contributing factor to heart disease, and a well-functioning immune system helps to mitigate this risk.

6.Enhances Cognitive Function: Adequate sleep is crucial for cognitive function, including memory, attention, and decision-making. This can indirectly benefit heart health by promoting healthy behaviors and choices, like maintaining a balanced diet and engaging in regular physical activity.

7. Optimizes Recovery and Repair: During sleep, the body undergoes essential repair and recovery processes. This includes the repair of damaged cells, tissues, and muscles. This restoration is vital for overall health and well being, including the health of the cardiovascular system.

8. Reduces Inflammation: Chronic inflammation is a major contributor to heart disease. Quality sleep helps to regulate inflammation levels in the body. When you're well-rested, the body is better equipped to manage inflammation, reducing the risk of heart-related issues.

9. Enhances Mental Health: Adequate sleep is crucial for maintaining good mental health. Conditions like depression and anxiety, if left untreated, can contribute to heart disease. Getting enough rest supports mental wellbeing, indirectly benefiting heart health.

10. Optimizes Endothelial Function: Sleep has been shown to improve endothelial function, which is the ability of blood vessels to expand and contract properly. Healthy endothelial function is crucial for good circulation and overall heart health.

11. Improves Mood and Emotional Well being: A good night's sleep is closely linked to improved mood and emotional stability. Positive mental health contributes to an overall sense of well being and can indirectly support a healthy heart lifestyle.

In conclusion, prioritizing adequate sleep and rest is an integral part of maintaining a healthy heart lifestyle. It plays a multifaceted role in regulating various physiological functions, reducing risk factors, and promoting overall well being. Incorporating good sleep habits into your routine can significantly contribute to a healthy heart and a higher quality of life.

Preventing heart diseases

Preventing heart diseases is of paramount importance in achieving and sustaining optimal health. As one of the leading causes of mortality worldwide, a proactive approach to heart health is essential for a long and fulfilling life. Understanding the key factors that contribute to cardiovascular health, adopting a balanced lifestyle, and making informed choices regarding diet, exercise, and stress management are all critical components of a comprehensive heart disease prevention strategy. This introductory paragraph sets the stage for a deeper exploration of the various measures and practices that can significantly reduce the risk of heart-related ailments, ultimately promoting a robust and resilient cardiovascular system.

Chapter 4

Preventing heart diseases

Smoking cessation is one of the most effective measures individuals can take to prevent heart diseases and improve overall cardiovascular health. The harmful effects of smoking on the heart and circulatory system are well-documented, and quitting smoking can lead to significant positive changes in a relatively short period. Here's an extensive look at how smoking cessation helps in preventing heart diseases:

Smoking cessation

1. Reduction in Cardiovascular Risk Factors:

Blood Pressure Regulation: Smoking raises blood pressure by causing the arteries to narrow and constrict. When a person quits smoking, blood pressure levels start to normalize, reducing the strain on the heart and lowering the risk of hypertension.

- Improvement in Cholesterol Levels: Smoking leads to lower levels of HDL (high-density lipoprotein) or "good" cholesterol and higher levels of LDL (low-density lipoprotein) or "bad" cholesterol. Quitting smoking helps to restore a healthier balance of these lipids, reducing the risk of plaque buildup in the arteries.

2. Enhanced Blood Circulation:

- Improved Endothelial Function: Smoking damages the endothelium, the inner lining of blood vessels, impairing its ability to expand and contract properly. After quitting, the endothelial function starts to recover, leading to better blood flow and overall cardiovascular health.

3. Reduced Risk of Atherosclerosis:

- Decreased Plaque Formation: Smoking accelerates the formation of fatty deposits (plaque) in the arteries, leading to atherosclerosis. By quitting, the progression of this condition is slowed down, reducing the risk of heart attacks and strokes.

4. Lowered Heart Rate and Carbon Monoxide Levels:

- Restoration of Normal Heart Rate: Smoking elevates heart rate by stimulating the release of adrenaline. After quitting, heart rate gradually returns to a healthier, more stable rhythm.

- Elimination of Carbon Monoxide: Smoking introduces carbon monoxide into the bloodstream, which competes with oxygen, reducing the amount of oxygen available for the heart and body tissues. Quitting smoking allows oxygen levels to normalize.

5. Improved Long-term Survival Rates:

- Decreased Mortality Risk: Studies consistently show that individuals who quit smoking have a significantly lower risk of dying from heart disease compared to those who continue to smoke. The benefits increase with each year of smoking cessation.

6. Reduction in Inflammation and Oxidative Stress:

- Lowered Inflammatory Markers: Smoking triggers chronic inflammation, a key contributor to heart disease. When a person quits, inflammatory markers decrease, reducing the overall inflammatory burden on the cardiovascular system.

- Decreased Oxidative Stress: Smoking leads to increased oxidative stress, which damages cells and tissues. Quitting smoking helps to reduce oxidative stress, allowing the body to repair and regenerate more effectively.

7. Improved Response to Medical Interventions:

- Enhanced Effectiveness of Medications: People who quit smoking often respond better to medications for conditions like high blood pressure and high cholesterol. This means that treatment strategies are likely to be more successful in a non-smoking individual.

8. Reduced Risk of Secondhand Smoke Exposure:

- Protection for Others: Quitting smoking not only benefits the individual but also protects those around them from the harmful effects of secondhand smoke, which is a known risk factor for heart disease.

In conclusion, smoking cessation is a powerful intervention for preventing heart diseases and improving cardiovascular health. The positive effects on blood pressure, cholesterol levels, blood circulation, and overall cardiovascular function are substantial and contribute to a significantly reduced risk of heart-related conditions. Choosing to quit smoking is a pivotal step towards a healthier, longer, and more fulfilling life.

Limiting Alcohol Intake

Limiting alcohol consumption is a crucial aspect of maintaining heart health and preventing a range of cardiovascular conditions. While moderate alcohol intake has been associated with certain benefits, excessive or heavy drinking can have detrimental effects on the heart and circulatory system. This comprehensive guide explores the relationship between alcohol consumption and heart health, detailing the potential benefits of moderation and highlighting the risks associated with excessive drinking.

Moderate Alcohol Consumption And Heart Health:

1. Cardio protective Effects: Moderate alcohol consumption, particularly of red wine, has been linked to certain cardio protective effects. This is primarily attributed to the presence of antioxidants like resveratrol, which may help improve heart health.

2. Increased Levels of "Good" Cholesterol: Moderate alcohol consumption, particularly of red wine, has been associated with higher levels of high-density lipoprotein (HDL) cholesterol, often referred to as "good" cholesterol. Higher levels of HDL cholesterol can have a protective effect on the heart.

3. Improved Blood Flow: Some studies suggest that moderate alcohol consumption may lead to improved blood flow and circulation. This effect is thought to be related to the relaxation of blood vessels.

4. Reduced Risk of Ischemic Heart Disease: Moderate alcohol consumption has been linked to a reduced risk of ischemic heart disease, which is a condition characterized by reduced blood flow to the heart muscle.

Risks Of Excessive Alcohol Consumption:

1. Hypertension (High Blood Pressure): Excessive alcohol intake is a known risk factor for hypertension. It can lead to elevated blood pressure levels, which is a significant contributor to heart disease.

2. Arrhythmias and Cardiomyopathy: Heavy drinking can lead to irregular heart rhythms (arrhythmias) and weaken the heart muscle (cardiomyopathy), increasing the risk of heart failure.

3. Increased Risk of Stroke: Excessive alcohol consumption is associated with an elevated risk of stroke, which can result from high blood pressure, irregular heart rhythms, or the formation of blood clots.

4. Risk of Heart Failure: Chronic heavy drinking can lead to alcoholic cardiomyopathy, a condition where the heart muscle becomes weakened and enlarged, impairing its ability to pump blood effectively.

5. Impact on Cholesterol Levels: While moderate alcohol intake may increase "good" cholesterol levels, excessive consumption can lead to adverse effects on blood lipids, including elevated triglycerides.

6. Weight Gain and Obesity: Alcohol is calorie-dense, and excessive consumption can contribute to weight gain and obesity, both of which are risk factors for heart disease.

7. Liver Disease and Its Effects on the Heart: Chronic alcohol abuse can lead to liver disease, which in turn can affect the heart due to altered metabolism and impaired detoxification processes.

Individual Variations and Considerations:

It's important to note that individual responses to alcohol can vary, and what may be considered moderate for one person could be excessive for another. Additionally, the potential benefits of moderate alcohol consumption must be weighed against the risks, especially for individuals with a history of alcohol-related problems or those at higher risk for heart disease.

Conclusion:

While moderate alcohol consumption may offer some potential benefits for heart health, these benefits must be weighed against the well-documented risks of excessive drinking. For those concerned about their heart health, it is crucial to consult with a healthcare provider to assess individual risk factors and make informed decisions regarding alcohol consumption. Ultimately, maintaining a balanced and healthy lifestyle, including limiting alcohol intake, is a cornerstone of preventing heart diseases and promoting overall well being.

Managing Blood Sugar And Cholesterol

Overseeing pulse and cholesterol levels is central for keeping up with cardiovascular well being and forestalling heart infections. Both hypertension (hypertension) and raised cholesterol levels are significant gamble factors for heart-related conditions. This thorough aide will dive into different parts of circulatory strain and cholesterol the board, including way of life adjustments, dietary decisions, and clinical mediations.

Overseeing Blood Pressure:

1. Way Of Life Modifications:

- Normal Exercise: Participating in customary actual work assists with keeping a solid weight, reinforce the heart, and further develop vein capability. High-impact practices like strolling, running, and swimming are especially useful.

- Dietary Changes: Embracing an eating regimen wealthy in natural products, vegetables, entire grains, and lean proteins while diminishing sodium admission can essentially bring down circulatory strain. The Scramble (Dietary Ways to deal with Stop

Hypertension) diet is explicitly intended to assist with overseeing pulse.

- Stress Decrease Techniques: Rehearsing unwinding strategies like profound breathing, contemplation, and yoga can assist with bringing down feelings of anxiety, which thusly can decidedly affect circulatory strain.

- **Restricting Liquor and Caffeine**: Over the top utilization of liquor and caffeine can prompt raised pulse. Control is key in the two cases.

2. Medications:

- Anti hypertensive Medications: In situations where way of life adjustments alone are lacking, medical services suppliers might endorse drugs to assist with bringing down circulatory strain. These may incorporate diuretics, beta-blockers, ACE inhibitors, and calcium channel blockers, among others.

3.Ordinary Monitoring:

- Home Pulse Monitoring: Monitoring circulatory strain at home can give significant data and assist people and medical care suppliers with pursuing informed choices in regards to therapy plans.

Overseeing Cholesterol Levels:

1. Way of life Modifications:

- Heart-Solid Diet: Taking on an eating regimen low in immersed and trans fats, and high in fiber, organic products, vegetables, and entire grains can assist with bringing down cholesterol levels. Food varieties like greasy fish, nuts, and olive oil, which are wealthy in omega-3 unsaturated fats, can likewise be valuable.
- Normal Exercise: Actual work helps raise "great" HDL cholesterol and lower "terrible" LDL cholesterol. Go for the gold 150 minutes of moderate-power practice each week.
- Weight Management: Accomplishing and keeping a solid weight can decidedly influence cholesterol levels.

2. Medications:

- Statins and Other Lipid-Bringing down Drugs: At the point when way of life alterations alone are inadequate, medical care suppliers might endorse drugs like statins to bring down cholesterol levels. These meds work by diminishing the development of cholesterol in the liver.

3. Ordinary Monitoring:

- Cholesterol Testing: Ordinary blood tests can give vital data about cholesterol levels. It's critical to screen both LDL and HDL cholesterol levels, as well as fatty substances.

4. Smoking Cessation:

- Stopping smoking is fundamental for overseeing cholesterol levels. Smoking brings down "great" HDL cholesterol yet in addition harms veins, making them more helpless to the development of plaque.

Cooperation with Medical services Providers:

Normal check-ups and open correspondence with medical care suppliers are vital for powerful pulse and cholesterol the board. They can offer customized guidance, screen headway, and make changes in accordance with treatment plans depending on the situation.

Conclusion:

Overseeing circulatory strain and cholesterol levels is a multi-layered try that requires a mix of way of life changes, meds, and normal checking. By embracing heart-solid propensities and working intimately with medical care suppliers, people can essentially decrease their gamble of heart illnesses and partake in a greater of life. Keep in mind, consistency and obligation to these actions are critical to long haul cardiovascular wellbeing.

Chapter 5

Recognizing early signs of heart problems

Recognizing early signs of heart problems is crucial for maintaining cardiovascular health and preventing potentially serious complications. These indicators can vary widely, from subtle discomfort to more pronounced symptoms. Being attuned to changes in your body, understanding risk factors, and seeking medical attention promptly can make a significant difference in the early detection and management of heart-related issues. This knowledge empowers individuals to take proactive steps towards a heart-healthy lifestyle, ultimately reducing the risk of heart disease and its associated complications.

Common Symptoms Of Heart Issue

Certainly, recognizing common symptoms of heart issues is essential for early intervention and effective treatment. Here are some of the most prevalent signs to be aware of:

1.Chest Pain or Discomfort: This is often the most prominent symptom of a heart problem. It can manifest as a tightness, pressure, squeezing, or burning sensation in the chest. It may also radiate to the arms, neck, jaw, or back.

2.Shortness of Breath: If you experience difficulty in breathing, especially during physical activity or when lying down, it could be indicative of a heart issue. This symptom may be accompanied by a feeling of suffocation or tightness in the chest.

3. Fatigue: Unexplained and excessive tiredness or fatigue can be a sign of heart trouble. This fatigue may be particularly noticeable during everyday activities or exercise.

4.Rapid or Irregular Heartbeat (Palpitations): Sensations of a fluttering or pounding heart, or a sensation of irregular heartbeat, can indicate an underlying heart issue. It may feel like your heart is racing, skipping beats, or beating too slowly.

5. Dizziness or Lightheaded: Feeling dizzy or lightheaded, especially when standing up quickly, may be a sign that your heart is not pumping blood effectively.

6.Swelling (Edema): Fluid retention leading to swelling in the legs, ankles, feet, or abdomen can be an indication of heart failure or other cardiovascular issues.

7.Coughing or Wheezing: Persistent coughing or wheezing, particularly when lying down or at night, may be due to fluid accumulation in the lungs, which can be a symptom of heart failure.

8. Nausea or Loss of Appetite: Some people with heart issues may experience a feeling of queasiness, indigestion, or a loss of appetite. This can be a result of reduced blood flow to the digestive system.

9.Cold Sweat: Experiencing sudden, cold, clammy sweats without any apparent reason can be a symptom of heart problems, especially during a heart attack.

10. Cyanosis (Bluish Tint to Skin): In more severe cases, a bluish tint to the lips, fingers, or extremities can be a sign of reduced oxygen levels in the blood, which may be linked to heart issues.

It is important to note that not everyone experiencing heart issues will display all of these symptoms, and the severity and combination of symptoms can vary widely. Additionally, some individuals, particularly women, may experience atypical symptoms like discomfort in the neck, back, or jaw, or nausea and vomiting without chest pain. If you experience any of these symptoms, especially if they are sudden or severe, seeking immediate medical attention is crucial. Early detection and intervention can significantly improve outcomes for individuals with heart issues.

When to seek medical attention

Recognizing early signs of heart problems is crucial for timely intervention and preventing potentially serious complications. It's important to note that I'm not a doctor, but I can offer some general guidance. If you suspect you or someone else may be experiencing symptoms related to heart issues, it is always best to consult a healthcare professional for proper assessment and advice.

1. Chest Pain or Discomfort: This is one of the most common early signs of heart problems. It may feel like a tightness, pressure, fullness, or squeezing sensation in the chest. The pain may also radiate to the arms, neck, jaw, shoulder blades, or back.

2.Shortness of Breath: If you find it difficult to breathe or experience breathlessness during normal activities or at rest, it could be a sign of heart trouble. This symptom may occur with or without chest discomfort.

3. Fatigue and Weakness: Feeling unusually tired, even after adequate rest, could be indicative of an underlying heart issue. If you find yourself exhausted after minimal exertion, it's worth seeking medical attention.

4.Rapid or Irregular Heartbeat (Palpitations): Sensing your heart racing, fluttering, or experiencing irregular beats can be a sign of an arrhythmia or other heart condition.

5.Dizziness or Fainting: Sudden episodes of dizziness, lightheadedness, or fainting can be related to heart problems. If you experience these symptoms, especially in combination with other signs, it's important to consult a healthcare professional.

6. Swelling (Edema): Fluid retention, particularly in the legs, ankles, and feet, can be a sign of heart failure. This occurs when the heart is unable to pump blood effectively.

7. Coughing or Wheezing: Persistent coughing, especially if it produces pink, frothy sputum, may be indicative of heart failure. It's important to consult a healthcare provider to rule out cardiac involvement.

8. Cyanosis (Bluish Tinge to Lips and Fingertips): This can be a sign of poor circulation or oxygenation, which can be related to heart problems.

9. Chest Discomfort during Physical Activity: If you experience chest pain, tightness, or discomfort during exercise or physical exertion, it's a warning sign that requires immediate attention.

10.Excessive Sweating: Profuse sweating, especially when accompanied by other symptoms like chest pain or shortness of breath, may be a sign of a heart issue.

11. Nausea or Vomiting: While not as common, some people may experience nausea or vomiting as a result of heart problems, particularly during a heart attack.

12. Unexplained Weight Gain: Rapid and unexplained weight gain can be associated with heart failure, due to fluid retention.

Remember, these symptoms can vary from person to person, and some individuals may experience heart problems without any obvious warning signs. It's important to trust your instincts and seek medical attention if you have concerns about your heart health. If you or someone you know is experiencing severe symptoms like chest pain, difficulty breathing, or loss of consciousness, don't hesitate to call emergency services immediately.

Chapter 6

Medical Test And Screening

Medical tests and screenings play a crucial role in assessing and monitoring an individual's health status. These diagnostic procedures encompass a wide range of techniques, from simple physical examinations to sophisticated laboratory analyses and imaging studies. They serve as invaluable tools for healthcare professionals to detect, diagnose, and monitor various medical conditions, enabling timely intervention and effective treatment. By providing objective data about a patient's physiological state, these tests serve as a cornerstone in modern medicine, aiding in the formulation of accurate diagnoses and personalized treatment plans. This introductory paragraph sets the stage for a comprehensive exploration of the significance and diversity of medical tests and screenings in healthcare.

Routine Heart Health Check Up

Routine heart health check-ups are fundamental components of preventive healthcare, aimed at assessing and managing cardiovascular well-being. These regular evaluations are crucial in identifying risk factors, detecting early signs of heart disease, and implementing preventive measures to mitigate potential complications. Typically conducted by primary care physicians or cardiologists, these check-ups encompass a range of assessments, including medical history review, physical examinations, and various diagnostic tests.

One of the initial steps in a routine heart health check-up involves a detailed discussion of the patient's medical history. This encompasses information about past illnesses, family history of heart disease, lifestyle habits, and any existing cardiovascular risk factors such as hypertension, diabetes, or high cholesterol levels. Understanding this background provides a foundation for tailoring the check-up to the individual's specific health profile.

Physical examinations are a crucial aspect of these check-ups. Physicians evaluate vital signs like blood pressure, heart rate, and respiratory rate, which offer valuable insights into cardiovascular health. Additionally, they may listen to the heart sounds using a stethoscope to detect any abnormal rhythms or murmurs, which can indicate underlying heart conditions. The examination may also involve assessing peripheral pulses and examining for signs of fluid retention or swelling, which could be indicative of heart failure or other circulatory issues.

In addition to the history review and physical examination, routine heart health check-ups often incorporate a battery of diagnostic tests. One of the most common tests is an electrocardiogram (ECG or EKG), which records the electrical activity of the heart over a period of time. This helps identify irregularities in heart rhythm and can provide vital information on conditions like arrhythmias or ischemia.

Furthermore, lipid profile assessments are performed to measure cholesterol levels, including high-density lipoprotein (HDL) and low-density lipoprotein (LDL) cholesterol, as well as triglycerides. Elevated levels of LDL cholesterol are a significant risk factor for atherosclerosis and coronary artery disease, making this test an essential component of heart health evaluations.

Another important diagnostic tool in routine heart health check-ups is a stress test. This involves monitoring the heart's response to physical exertion, typically through treadmill exercises or medication-induced stress. It provides valuable information on how the heart functions under increased demand, aiding in the detection of ischemic heart disease.

Depending on the individual's risk factors and specific health concerns, additional tests like echocardiography (ultrasound imaging of the heart), coronary calcium scoring, or ambulatory blood pressure monitoring may be recommended. These supplementary assessments offer more comprehensive insights into heart structure, function, and overall cardiovascular health.

In conclusion, routine heart health check-ups are a cornerstone of preventive healthcare, serving as a proactive approach to maintaining cardiovascular well-being. Through a comprehensive evaluation of medical history, physical examination, and an array of diagnostic tests, healthcare professionals can identify potential risk factors and early signs of heart disease. Timely intervention and lifestyle modifications based on the findings of these check-ups can significantly reduce the likelihood of developing serious cardiovascular conditions, ultimately promoting a longer, healthier life. It is imperative for individuals to prioritize and engage in regular heart health assessments as a proactive measure towards maintaining optimal cardiac well-being.

Diagnostic Tests For Heart Condition

Certainly! Diagnostic tests for heart health play a crucial role in assessing the function and condition of the heart. They help healthcare professionals detect and monitor various heart-related conditions, ranging from coronary artery disease to arrhythmias. Here are some of the commonly used diagnostic tests for heart health:

1. Electrocardiogram (ECG or EKG): This is a non-invasive test that records the electrical activity of the heart over a period of time. Electrodes are placed on the skin, and the ECG machine produces a graph (ECG tracing) that shows the heart's rhythm and electrical activity. It can help identify irregularities in heart rhythm, signs of a heart attack, and other heart conditions.

2. Echocardiogram: This is an ultrasound test that uses high-frequency sound waves to create images of the heart's structure, valves, and blood flow. It provides information about the size, shape, and pumping function of the heart. Echocardiograms are useful for diagnosing conditions like heart valve problems, heart muscle diseases, and congenital heart defects.

3. Stress Test: This test evaluates how well your heart functions during physical activity. It typically involves walking on a treadmill or using medication to simulate the effects of exercise. During the test, your heart rate, blood pressure, and ECG are monitored. It can help diagnose coronary artery disease and assess the effectiveness of treatment.

4. Holter Monitor: This is a portable device that continuously records the heart's electrical activity over a 24 to 48-hour period. It is typically used for patients who experience intermittent symptoms like palpitations or dizziness. The data captured helps identify irregular heart rhythms that may not be detected during a standard ECG.

5. Cardiac Catheterization (Coronary Angiography): This is an invasive procedure where a thin, flexible tube (catheter) is inserted into a blood vessel in the arm or groin and threaded to the heart. Contrast dye is then injected, and X-ray images are taken to visualize the coronary arteries. It is used to identify blockages or narrowing of the arteries and to guide treatment options like angioplasty or stent placement.

6. Computed Tomography (CT) Angiography: This is a non-invasive imaging test that uses X-rays and computer technology to create detailed cross-sectional images of the heart and blood vessels. It is particularly useful for assessing the presence and extent of coronary artery disease.

7. MRI (Magnetic Resonance Imaging): Cardiac MRI uses strong magnetic fields and radio waves to create detailed images of the heart. It provides information about the heart's structure, function, and blood flow. MRI is helpful in diagnosing a wide range of heart conditions, including congenital heart defects and heart muscle disorders.

8. Blood Tests: Various blood tests can provide valuable information about heart health. For example, a lipid profile measures cholesterol levels, and high levels of LDL cholesterol are associated with an increased risk of heart disease. Other blood tests can assess levels of cardiac enzymes or biomarkers that indicate heart muscle damage, such as troponin and creatine kinase.

It's important to note that the choice of diagnostic test(s) will depend on the individual's symptoms, medical history, and risk factors. A healthcare provider will recommend specific tests based on their assessment of the patient's condition. Always consult a healthcare professional for personalized advice and interpretation of test results.

Chapter 7

Treatment Options For Heart Condition

Treatment options for heart conditions encompass a diverse array of interventions aimed at managing and improving the health of the cardiovascular system. From lifestyle modifications to advanced medical procedures, these approaches are tailored to address a wide spectrum of cardiac issues, including coronary artery disease, heart failure, arrhythmias, and valvular disorders. The selection of an appropriate treatment plan hinges on factors such as the specific diagnosis, the severity of the condition, and the patient's overall health. In this context, healthcare providers may recommend lifestyle changes, medications, interventional procedures, or, in more complex cases, surgical interventions. This introductory paragraph provides a glimpse into the multifaceted nature of heart disease treatment, reflecting the importance of personalized care to optimize cardiac health and enhance overall well-being

Medication For Heart Health

Certainly! Medications play a crucial role in the management of various heart conditions. They can help control symptoms, develop heart function, and reduce the risk of complications. Here is an extensive overview of some common classes of medications used for heart health:

1. Anticoagulants and Antiplatelet Drugs:

   - *Warfarin, Apixaban, Rivaroxaban, Dabigatran:*These drugs are anticoagulants, also known as blood thinners. They help prevent blood clots from forming or getting larger. They are used to treat conditions like atrial fibrillation, deep vein thrombosis, and pulmonary embolism.

   - Aspirin, Clopidogrel, Prasugrel: These are antiplatelet drugs that prevent blood cells (platelets) from sticking together and forming clots. They are often prescribed after a heart attack, stroke, or in cases of coronary artery disease.

2. ACE Inhibitors (Angiotensin-Converting Enzyme Inhibitors):

- Enalapril, Lisinopril, Ramipril: ACE inhibitors relax blood vessels and lower blood pressure. They are commonly used to treat conditions like hypertension, heart failure, and diabetic kidney disease.

3. ARBs (Angiotensin II Receptor Blockers):

- Losartan, Valsartan, Irbesartan: Similar to ACE inhibitors, ARBs also help relax blood vessels and lower blood pressure. They are often prescribed for patients who cannot tolerate ACE inhibitors due to side effects.

4. Beta Blockers:
- Metoprolol, Atenolol, Carvedilol: Beta blockers reduce the heart rate and decrease the force of contractions, which can help lower blood pressure and reduce the workload on the heart. They are commonly used to treat conditions like hypertension, angina, and heart failure.

5. Calcium Channel Blockers:
- Amlodipine, Verapamil, Diltiazem: These drugs relax and widen blood vessels, which can help improve blood flow and lower

blood pressure. They are used to treat conditions like hypertension, angina, and certain arrhythmias.

6. Diuretics:

-Furosemide,Hydrochlorothiazide, Spironolactone: Diuretics help remove excess sodium and water from the body, which can help lower blood pressure and reduce the workload on the heart. They are commonly used to treat hypertension and heart failure.

7. Statins:

- Atorvastatin, Simvastatin, Rosuvastatin: Statins are used to lower cholesterol levels in the blood. They work by inhibiting an enzyme involved in cholesterol production. They are crucial in reducing the risk of atherosclerosis and coronary artery disease.

8. Nitrates:

- Nitroglycerin, Isosorbide dinitrate: Nitrates relax and widen blood vessels, improving blood flow to the heart muscle. They are used to treat angina (chest pain) and heart failure.

9. Digitalis Preparations:

- Digoxin: This medication helps strengthen the heart's contractions and regulate its rhythm. It is used primarily in cases of heart failure and certain types of arrhythmias.

10. Antiarrhythmic Drugs:

- Amiodarone, Flecainide, Sotalol: These medications are used to regulate and stabilize heart rhythm in cases of arrhythmias.

It's important to note that medication management should be personalized, and patients should follow their healthcare provider's instructions carefully. Additionally, regular monitoring and follow-up appointments are essential to ensure the effectiveness and safety of the prescribed medications. Always consult a healthcare professional for specific advice regarding medications for heart health.

Surgical And Interventional Procedures

Surgical and interventional procedures are essential components of heart disease treatment. They range from minimally invasive interventions to complex surgeries, each tailored to address specific cardiac conditions. Here is an extensive overview of some common surgical and interventional procedures used in heart health:

1. Coronary Artery Bypass Grafting (CABG):

- Description: CABG, often referred to as "bypass surgery," is a major surgical procedure used to treat severe coronary artery disease. It involves rerouting blood flow around blocked or narrowed coronary arteries using grafts (usually from the patient's own veins or arteries) to restore blood supply to the heart muscle.

- Indications: Severe coronary artery disease, particularly when multiple arteries are affected.

2. Percutaneous Coronary Intervention (PCI) / Angioplasty:

- Description: PCI is a minimally invasive procedure used to open narrowed or blocked coronary arteries. A catheter with a balloon at its tip is threaded through a blood vessel to the site of the blockage. The balloon is inflated to compress the plaque, and a stent may be placed to keep the artery open.

- Indications: Acute heart attacks, unstable angina, and significant coronary artery blockages.

3. Stent Placement:

- Description: Stents are small mesh tubes that can be inserted during an angioplasty. They are placed in the narrowed coronary artery to help keep it open and maintain blood flow.

- Indications: Used in conjunction with angioplasty for patients with coronary artery disease.

4. Valve Repair or Replacement:

- Description: This surgical procedure involves repairing or replacing damaged heart valves. Valves can be repaired by reconstructing the valve tissue or repairing leaflets, while replacement involves replacing the valve with a mechanical or biological prosthesis.

- Indications: Valve stenosis (narrowing) or regurgitation (leaking), which can be due to conditions like aortic stenosis or mitral valve prolapse.

5. Ablation Therapy:

- Description: Ablation is a minimally invasive procedure used to treat certain types of abnormal heart rhythms (arrhythmias). It involves using heat or cold energy to destroy the tissue that is causing the abnormal electrical signals in the heart.

- Indications: Atrial fibrillation, supra ventricular tachycardia, and other arrhythmias.

6. Pacemaker Implantation:

- Description: A pacemaker is a small electronic device that is implanted under the skin, usually near the collarbone. It helps regulate the heart's rhythm by sending electrical impulses to the heart muscle, ensuring a steady heartbeat.

- Indications: Bradycardia (slow heart rate) and certain types of arrhythmias.

7. Implantable Cardioverter Defibrillator (ICD) Placement:

- Description: Similar to a pacemaker, an ICD is a device implanted under the skin. It continuously monitors the heart's rhythm and can deliver electric shocks to restore normal rhythm in the event of a dangerous arrhythmia or sudden cardiac arrest.

- Indications: High-risk patients with a history of life-threatening arrhythmias or cardiac arrest.

8. Heart Transplant:

- Description: A heart transplant is a complex surgical procedure in which a diseased or failing heart is replaced with a healthy heart from a deceased donor. It is reserved for patients with end-stage heart failure when other treatments have been unsuccessful.

- Indications: Severe heart failure that is unresponsive to other treatment options.

9. Ventricular Assist Device (VAD) Implantation:

- Description: A VAD is a mechanical pump that is surgically implanted to assist a weakened heart in pumping blood. It is used as a bridge to transplant or as a destination therapy for patients who are not transplant candidates.

- Indications: Severe heart failure when transplant is not immediately available.

10. Minimally Invasive Procedures:

- Description: These procedures use small incisions and specialized instruments to access and treat the heart. Examples include minimally invasive valve repair or replacement and certain types of ablation procedures.

   - Indications: Selected cases where less invasive options are suitable.

These surgical and interventional procedures are carried out by highly skilled cardiac surgeons and interventional cardiologists in specialized medical centers. The choice of procedure depends on the specific diagnosis, the patient's overall health, and the expertise of the medical team. It's important for patients to discuss their options thoroughly with their healthcare providers and to weigh the potential benefits and risks of each procedure.

Life Style Modification In Treatment

Lifestyle modifications are a cornerstone of heart health and play a pivotal role in preventing and managing various cardiovascular conditions. These changes, when adopted consistently, can significantly improve heart function, reduce risk factors, and enhance overall well-being. Here is an extensive overview of key lifestyle modifications for heart health:

1. Healthy Diet:

- Balanced Nutrition: A heart-healthy diet emphasizes whole, nutrient-dense foods such as fruits, vegetables, whole grains, lean proteins, and healthy fats. It limits the intake of processed foods, saturated and trans fats, excessive salt, and added sugars.

- Portion Control: Paying attention to portion sizes helps maintain a healthy weight and prevents over consumption of calories.

2. Regular Exercise:

- Aerobic Activities: Engaging in regular aerobic exercise, such as brisk walking, jogging, swimming, or cycling, helps improve cardiovascular fitness, lower blood pressure, and manage weight.

- **Strength Training:** Incorporating strength-building exercises, like weightlifting or resistance training, helps improve muscle tone, metabolism, and overall physical function.

3. Maintain a Healthy Weight:

- Achieving and maintaining a healthy body weight reduces the strain on the heart and lowers the risk of conditions like high blood pressure, diabetes, and high cholesterol.

4. Smoking Cessation:

- Quitting smoking is one of the most impactful steps towards better heart health. Smoking damages blood vessels, increases blood pressure, and raises the risk of heart disease.

5. Limit Alcohol Intake:

- Excessive alcohol consumption can contribute to high blood pressure, irregular heart rhythms, and heart muscle damage. Moderation or abstaining from alcohol is advised.

6. Stress Management:

- Mindfulness and Relaxation Techniques: Practices like meditation, deep breathing exercises, yoga, and progressive muscle relaxation can help reduce stress levels.
- Regular Physical Activity: Exercise is not only beneficial for physical health but also helps alleviate stress by releasing endorphins, the body's natural mood elevators.

7. Adequate Sleep:

- Getting 7-9 hours of quality sleep per night supports overall health, including heart health. Poor sleep patterns have been associated with increased risk of heart disease.

8. Regular Health Check-ups:

- Regular visits to a healthcare provider for check-ups, blood pressure monitoring, cholesterol checks, and diabetes management are crucial for early detection and management of risk factors.

9. Medication Adherence:

- Following prescribed medications and treatment plans as directed by healthcare providers is essential for managing conditions like hypertension, high cholesterol, and diabetes.

10. Limiting Processed Foods and Added Sugars:

- Processed foods, which often contain excessive sodium, unhealthy fats, and added sugars, should be limited. Opting for whole, minimally processed foods is a healthier choice.

11. Hydration:

- Staying well-hydrated supports overall health. Water is crucial for proper circulation and helps maintain blood pressure.

12. Regular Monitoring and Self-awareness:

- Being aware of one's own health indicators, like blood pressure, cholesterol levels, and body weight, empowers individuals to take proactive steps towards better heart health.

It's important to note that lifestyle modifications are not a one-size-fits-all approach. They should be personalized based on individual health status, medical history, and specific cardiovascular risk factors. Additionally, making these changes gradually and seeking guidance from healthcare providers or registered dietitians can help ensure a sustainable and effective approach to heart health. Remember, consistency and commitment to these lifestyle modifications can lead to significant improvements in heart health and overall quality of life.

Chapter 8

Cardiac Rehabilitation And Recovery

Cardiac rehabilitation and recovery form a pivotal phase in the journey of individuals who have experienced heart-related events or undergone cardiac procedures. This comprehensive program is designed to support and guide patients through the process of healing, both physically and emotionally. It encompasses a range of structured interventions, including tailored exercise regimens, educational sessions, counseling, and lifestyle modifications. The primary objectives of cardiac rehabilitation are to optimize cardiovascular health, reduce the risk of future heart-related issues, and enhance overall well-being. By providing a holistic approach to recovery, cardiac rehabilitation empowers individuals to take an active role in their health, enabling them to lead fulfilling and heart-healthy lives. This introductory phase sets the foundation for a journey towards improved heart health and a brighter, more vibrant future.

Post Treatment Care And Rehabilitation

Post-treatment care and rehabilitation are critical phases in the continuum of care for individuals who have undergone cardiac interventions or experienced heart-related events. These phases focus on ensuring optimal recovery, minimizing complications, and promoting long-term heart health. Here is an extensive overview of post-treatment care and rehabilitation:

1.Medical Follow-Up:

- Regular Check-Ups: After a cardiac event or procedure, individuals should have regular follow-up appointments with their healthcare provider. These visits are crucial for monitoring progress, assessing risk factors, and adjusting treatment plans as needed.

- Medication Management: Ensuring adherence to prescribed medications and monitoring for any side effects or interactions is essential for maintaining heart health.

2. Diet and Nutrition:

- Heart-Healthy Eating: Continuing a heart-healthy diet, rich in fruits, vegetables, whole grains, lean proteins, and healthy fats, is crucial for managing cholesterol levels, blood pressure, and overall heart health.

- Portion Control: Practicing portion control helps maintain a healthy weight and prevents over consumption of calories.

3. Physical Activity and Exercise:

- Gradual Resumption of Activity: After receiving clearance from healthcare providers, individuals should gradually resume physical activities. This may include walking, light aerobic exercises, and gradually increasing intensity.

- Structured Exercise Programs: Participation in a cardiac rehabilitation program or supervised exercise regimen can help individuals safely rebuild cardiovascular fitness under the guidance of trained professionals.

4. Lifestyle Modifications:

- Smoking Cessation: Continuing to abstain from smoking is crucial for long-term heart health. Support programs and resources for smoking cessation should be readily available.

- Moderate Alcohol Consumption: If alcohol is consumed, it should be done in moderation, as excessive intake can contribute to heart-related issues.

5. Stress Management:

- Stress-Reduction Techniques: Implementing stress-reduction techniques such as meditation, deep breathing exercises, and mindfulness practices can help improve mental and emotional well-being.

- Engagement in Relaxing Activities: Engaging in hobbies, spending time with loved ones, and participating in activities that bring joy and relaxation are important for managing stress.

6. Psycho social Support:

- Counseling and Support Groups: Emotional well-being is integral to overall recovery. Participation in counseling or support groups can help individuals navigate the emotional impact of a cardiac event and build a strong support network.

7. Continued Education:

- Health Literacy: Ongoing education about heart health, risk factors, and self-care measures empowers individuals to actively manage their cardiovascular health.

- Understanding Warning Signs: Knowing the signs of a potential cardiac event and when to seek immediate medical attention is crucial for early intervention.

8. Long-Term Risk Management:

- Blood Pressure and Cholesterol Control:Regular monitoring and management of blood pressure and cholesterol levels are vital for preventing future heart-related issues.
- Diabetes Management: For individuals with diabetes, maintaining stable blood sugar levels through diet, exercise, and medication management is essential for heart health.

9.Regular Medical Screenings:

- Screening Tests: Routine screenings for conditions like diabetes, high blood pressure, and high cholesterol are important for early detection and management.

10. Maintaining a Support System:

- Family and Social Support: Having a strong support system of family, friends, and healthcare providers can provide emotional and practical support during the recovery process.

Post-treatment care and rehabilitation aim to optimize recovery, enhance quality of life, and reduce the risk of future heart-related issues. It is crucial for individuals to actively participate in their own care and to communicate any concerns or changes in health status with their healthcare providers. With consistent adherence to post-treatment care and rehabilitation guidelines, individuals can achieve long-lasting heart health and well-being.

Emotional Well Being And Support

Emotional well-being and support are integral components of holistic healthcare, particularly for individuals navigating heart-related events or cardiac interventions. Addressing the emotional aspect of recovery is essential, as it can significantly impact overall well-being and the success of rehabilitation efforts. Here is an extensive overview of emotional well-being and support in the context of heart health:

1. Impact of Emotional Health on Heart Health:

- Bidirectional Relationship: There is a complex interplay between emotional well-being and heart health. Chronic stress, anxiety, depression, and other negative emotions can contribute to the development or exacerbation of heart conditions, while heart-related events or diagnoses can have a profound impact on emotional well-being.

2. Common Emotional Responses:

- Anxiety and Fear: Individuals may experience heightened anxiety and fear, particularly after a heart-related event or procedure. This can be related to concerns about future health, lifestyle changes, and uncertainties about the recovery process.

- Depression: Feelings of sadness, hopelessness, and loss of interest or pleasure in activities are common in individuals with heart conditions. Depression can affect motivation for self-care and adherence to treatment plans.

3. Importance of Emotional Well-Being:

- Enhanced Quality of Life: Addressing emotional well-being leads to improved overall quality of life. It helps individuals cope with challenges, maintain social connections, and engage in activities that bring joy and fulfillment.

- Adherence to Treatment Plans: Emotional well-being is closely linked to adherence to medications, lifestyle modifications, and rehabilitation programs. When individuals feel supported and motivated, they are more likely to follow through with recommended treatments.

4. Strategies for Emotional Well-Being:

- Counseling and Therapy: Professional counseling or therapy, including cognitive behavioral therapy (CBT) and other evidence-based approaches, can help individuals address and manage emotional challenges.

-Mindfulness and Relaxation Techniques:Practices like meditation, deep breathing exercises, yoga, and progressive muscle relaxation can promote relaxation, reduce anxiety, and improve emotional well-being.

- Engagement in Enjoyable Activities: Pursuing hobbies, spending time with loved ones, and participating in activities that bring joy and relaxation contribute to emotional well-being.

- Open Communication: Sharing feelings, concerns, and questions with healthcare providers, family members, and support networks is crucial for receiving appropriate support and guidance.

5. Support Systems:

- Family and Friends: Strong social connections provide invaluable emotional support. Open communication with loved ones fosters understanding and empathy.

- Support Groups: Participating in support groups for individuals with heart conditions allows for shared experiences, mutual support, and a sense of belonging.

6. Psycho social Support in Cardiac Rehabilitation:

- Incorporation in Programs: Cardiac rehabilitation programs often include elements of psycho social support, such as counseling, stress management, and educational sessions on coping strategies.

7. Recognition and Management of Mental Health Conditions:

- Screening and Treatment: Identifying and addressing mental health conditions like anxiety and depression is crucial for overall well-being. This may involve consultation with mental health professionals and, in some cases, medication management.

8. Holistic Approach to Care:

- Collaborative Care: A multidisciplinary approach, involving healthcare providers, mental health professionals, and support networks, ensures that emotional well-being is integrated into the overall treatment plan.

9. Empowerment and Self-Care:

- Self-Advocacy: Empowering individuals to advocate for their emotional well-being, seek support, and communicate their needs is an important aspect of recovery.

Addressing emotional well-being alongside physical health is vital for comprehensive care in individuals with heart conditions. It promotes resilience, enhances coping mechanisms, and supports long-term heart health and overall quality of life. Encouraging open communication, providing access to mental health resources, and fostering a supportive environment are key elements in creating a holistic approach to heart health care.

Chapter 9

Living with a healthy heart

Living with a healthy heart is a trans-formative journey that encompasses not only physical well-being but also emotional and psychological vitality. It is a commitment to nurturing the cardiovascular system through mindful choices, balanced nutrition, regular exercise, and effective stress management. Embracing a heart-healthy lifestyle empowers individuals to proactively safeguard their cardiac health, reducing the risk of heart-related conditions and enhancing overall quality of life. This journey is marked by a harmonious fusion of nutritious habits, regular physical activity, and a supportive network of healthcare professionals and loved ones. Ultimately, living with a healthy heart paves the way for a life filled with vitality, resilience, and the promise of a brighter, more fulfilling future.

Long Term Heart Health Strategies

Long-term heart health strategies are essential for maintaining optimal cardiovascular well-being throughout one's lifetime. These strategies encompass a combination of lifestyle choices, regular medical check-ups, and ongoing management of risk factors. Here is an extensive overview of long-term heart health strategies:

1. Adopting a Heart-Healthy Lifestyle:

- Balanced Diet: Prioritize whole, nutrient-dense foods like fruits, vegetables, whole grains, lean proteins, and healthy fats. Minimize intake of processed foods, saturated and trans fats, excessive salt, and added sugars.
- Regular Exercise: Engage in regular aerobic activities, strength training, and flexibility exercises to improve cardiovascular fitness, muscle strength, and overall physical function.
- Avoiding Smoking and Excessive Alcohol:Quitting smoking and limiting alcohol consumption are crucial for long-term heart health. Smoking cessation programs and resources should be readily available.

2. Maintaining a Healthy Weight:

- Achieving and maintaining a healthy body weight reduces the strain on the heart and lowers the risk of conditions like high blood pressure, diabetes, and high cholesterol.

3. Regular Medical Check-ups:

- Blood Pressure Monitoring: Regular checks for high blood pressure are crucial for early detection and management.

- Cholesterol Screening: Routine assessments of cholesterol levels help identify and address high levels that may contribute to atherosclerosis.

- Diabetes Management: For individuals with diabetes, maintaining stable blood sugar levels is essential for heart health.

- Thorough Medical Evaluation: Regular visits to healthcare providers for comprehensive assessments of heart health, including ECGs, echo cardiograms, and other diagnostic tests, ensure early detection and management of potential issues.

4. Medication Adherence:

- Following prescribed medications and treatment plans as directed by healthcare providers is essential for managing conditions like hypertension, high cholesterol, and diabetes.

5. Stress Management:

-Mindfulness and Relaxation Techniques:Practices like meditation, deep breathing exercises, yoga, and progressive muscle relaxation can help reduce stress levels.

- Regular Physical Activity: Exercise is not only beneficial for physical health but also helps alleviate stress by releasing endorphins, the body's natural mood elevators.

6. Nutritional Guidance and Portion Control:

- Registered dietitians can provide personalized dietary recommendations to support heart-healthy eating habits. Monitoring portion sizes helps maintain a healthy weight and prevents overconsumption of calories.

7. Psycho social Support:

- Counseling and Support Groups: Emotional well-being is integral to long-term heart health. Participation in counseling or support groups can help individuals navigate the emotional impact of a cardiac event or ongoing heart condition.

8. Regular Exercise and Physical Activity:

- Lifetime Commitment: Engaging in regular physical activity should be a lifelong commitment. This may include a combination of aerobic activities, strength training, and flexibility exercises.

- Adapting to Age: Exercise routines may need to be adjusted over time to accommodate changing physical capabilities and needs.

9. Maintaining Social Connections:

- Strong Support Network: Building and maintaining strong social connections with family, friends, and support groups provides valuable emotional and practical support.

10. Continued Education and Health Literacy:

- Staying Informed: Ongoing education about heart health, risk factors, and self-care measures empowers individuals to actively manage their cardiovascular health.

11. Regular Screenings for Heart Conditions:

- Periodic screenings for conditions like high blood pressure, high cholesterol, and diabetes are important for early detection and management.

12. Consistent Communication with Healthcare Providers:

- Open and Proactive: Regular communication with healthcare providers about any changes in health status, concerns, or questions is crucial for receiving appropriate support and guidance.

Long-term heart health strategies are not only about preventing heart disease but also about thriving with optimal cardiovascular function throughout life. By embracing these strategies and maintaining a proactive approach to heart health, individuals can look forward to a vibrant and fulfilling future. It's important to remember that these strategies should be personalized based on individual health status and medical history, and should be discussed with a healthcare provider for tailored guidance.

Maintaining a Heart Healthy Lifestyle

Maintaining a heart-healthy lifestyle is a lifelong commitment to practices and choices that support optimal cardiovascular health. This approach involves a combination of balanced nutrition, regular physical activity, stress management, and avoiding risk factors. Here is an extensive overview of how to maintain a heart-healthy lifestyle:

1. Balanced Diet:

- Whole, Nutrient-Dense Foods: Prioritize a diet rich in fruits, vegetables, whole grains, lean proteins (such as poultry, fish, beans, and legumes), and healthy fats (like avocados, nuts, and olive oil).

- Limit Processed Foods: Minimize consumption of processed foods, which often contain excessive sodium, unhealthy fats, and added sugars.

2. Portion Control:

- Be mindful of portion sizes to prevent over consumption of calories and maintain a healthy weight.

3. Limit Saturated and Trans Fats:

- Sources of Saturated Fat: Limit foods high in saturated fats like red meat, full-fat dairy products, and fried or processed foods.
- Avoid Trans Fats: Minimize or avoid trans fats found in partially hydrogenated oils and many processed and packaged foods.

4. Reduce Sodium Intake:

- Aim to lower salt intake by choosing low-sodium options and minimizing the use of added salt in cooking.

5. Manage Cholesterol Levels:

- Include foods that help maintain healthy cholesterol levels, such as high-fiber foods, nuts, and foods rich in omega-3 fatty acids (like fatty fish).

6. Regular Physical Activity:

- Engage in regular aerobic activities like brisk walking, jogging, swimming, or cycling. Aim for at least 150 minutes of moderate-intensity exercise per week.

- Incorporate strength training exercises to improve muscle tone and metabolism.

7. Avoid Smoking and Excessive Alcohol:

- Smoking Cessation: Quitting smoking is one of the most impactful steps towards better heart health. Smoking damages blood vessels and increases the risk of heart disease.

- Moderate Alcohol Consumption: If alcohol is consumed, it should be done in moderation, as excessive intake can contribute to heart-related issues.

8. Maintain a Healthy Weight:

- Achieving and maintaining a healthy body weight is essential for reducing the risk of heart-related conditions.

9. Manage Stress:

- Mindfulness and Relaxation Techniques:Practices like meditation, deep breathing exercises, yoga, and progressive muscle relaxation can help reduce stress levels.

- Regular Exercise: Physical activity is an effective way to alleviate stress by releasing endorphins, the body's natural mood elevators.

10. Adequate Sleep:

- Aim for 7-9 hours of quality sleep per night to support overall health, including heart health.

11. Regular Health Check-ups:

- Routine visits to healthcare providers for check-ups, blood pressure monitoring, cholesterol checks, and diabetes management are crucial for early detection and management of risk factors.

12. Stay Informed and Educated:

- Learn about heart health, risk factors, and self-care measures to empower yourself in actively managing your cardiovascular health.

13. Seek Professional Guidance:

- Consult with healthcare providers or registered dietitians for personalized advice and guidance on maintaining a heart-healthy lifestyle.

14. Stay Hydrated:

- Drinking an adequate amount of water supports overall health, including proper circulation and maintenance of blood pressure.

15. Maintain a Positive Outlook:

- Cultivate a positive mindset and practice gratitude to promote mental and emotional well-being, which in turn supports heart health.

Maintaining a heart-healthy lifestyle is a multifaceted endeavor that requires commitment and consistency. It's important to remember that small, sustainable changes over time can have a significant impact on overall cardiovascular health. Consulting with healthcare providers for personalized guidance and regular check-ups is crucial for long-term success in maintaining a healthy heart.

Coping With Chronic Heart Condition

Coping with a chronic heart condition can be a significant challenge, both physically and emotionally. It requires a comprehensive approach that involves medical management, lifestyle adjustments, emotional support, and a proactive mindset. Here is an extensive overview of strategies for coping with a chronic heart condition:

1. Education and Understanding:
   - Empowerment Through Knowledge: Learning about your specific heart condition, its causes, symptoms, and treatment

options is crucial for making informed decisions and taking an active role in your care.

2. Open Communication with Healthcare Providers:
- Regular Check-Ups and Consultations:Maintaining a strong and open relationship with your healthcare team ensures that any changes in your condition are promptly addressed.

3. Adherence to Medical Recommendations:

- Medication Management: Taking prescribed medications as directed is essential for managing and controlling your heart condition.
- Follow Treatment Plans: This includes dietary restrictions, exercise routines, and other lifestyle modifications recommended by your healthcare provider.

4. Healthy Lifestyle Modifications:
- Balanced Diet: Embrace heart-healthy eating habits, focusing on whole, nutrient-dense foods and limiting processed and high-sodium foods.
- Regular Exercise: Engage in physical activity as recommended by your healthcare provider, tailored to your specific condition and capabilities.

5. Stress Management:

- Mindfulness and Relaxation Techniques:Practices like meditation, deep breathing exercises, yoga, and progressive muscle relaxation can help reduce stress levels.

- Engage in Relaxing Activities: Pursuing hobbies, spending time in nature, and participating in activities that bring joy and relaxation contribute to emotional well-being.

6. Psycho social Support:

- Counseling and Support Groups: Emotional well-being is integral to coping with a chronic heart condition. Participating in counseling or support groups can help you navigate the emotional impact of your condition and build a strong support network.

7. Monitor Your Condition:

- Awareness of Symptoms: Be vigilant about any changes in symptoms or new symptoms that may indicate a change in your condition. Report these to your healthcare provider promptly.

8. Adaptation and Flexibility:

- Adjusting to New Realities:Recognize that life may be different with a chronic heart condition. Adaptation may involve modifying activities, setting realistic goals, and finding new ways to stay engaged and active.

9. Seeking Emotional Support:

- Family and Friends: Lean on loved ones for emotional support and share your feelings and concerns. Open communication fosters understanding and empathy.

- Support Groups: Connecting with others who are experiencing similar challenges through support groups can provide a sense of community and shared experiences.

10. Maintaining a Positive Outlook:

- Cultivate a positive mindset and practice gratitude to promote mental and emotional well-being. A positive outlook can contribute to overall resilience in coping with a chronic heart condition.

11. Addressing Anxiety and Depression:

- Recognize and seek help for symptoms of anxiety or depression, which are common in individuals with chronic health conditions. Professional counseling or therapy may be beneficial.

12. Regular Health Screenings:

- Stay up-to-date with routine health screenings to monitor your heart health and identify any changes or potential complications.

13. Self-Advocacy:

- Advocate for your own health and communicate your needs and concerns to your healthcare team. Be an active participant in decisions about your care.

14. Celebrate Milestones and Achievements:

- Acknowledge and celebrate your accomplishments, whether they are related to managing your condition, achieving personal goals, or maintaining a positive outlook.

Coping with a chronic heart condition requires a holistic and proactive approach. It's important to remember that you are not alone, and there are resources and support available to help you navigate this journey. Regular communication with your healthcare team, maintaining a healthy lifestyle, and seeking emotional support are key components of effectively coping with a chronic heart condition.

Conclusion

In conclusion, the Heart Manual serves as an invaluable road map to a life of vibrant health and well-being. Its comprehensive guidance empowers individuals to take charge of their cardiovascular health through informed decisions and proactive lifestyle choices. By emphasizing the importance of balanced nutrition, regular exercise, stress management, and adherence to medical recommendations, this manual provides a solid foundation for maintaining a healthy heart.

Furthermore, the manual recognizes the intricate interplay between physical and emotional well-being, acknowledging that a holistic approach to health is paramount. It underscores the significance of open communication with healthcare providers, fostering a partnership that ensures personalized care and ongoing support. Additionally, the manual addresses the emotional impact of heart conditions, offering strategies for coping and seeking psycho social support.

Ultimately, the Heart Manual serves as a beacon of hope and empowerment for individuals on their journey to heart health. By following its clear and actionable guidance, one can not only mitigate the risk of heart-related issues but also cultivate a life filled with vitality, resilience, and the promise of a brighter, more fulfilling future. This manual stands as a testament to the potential for positive change and underscores the immense capacity individuals possess to lead a heart-healthy life.